Walking Alone Together

Pamela J. Klemm

DENVER, COLORADO

Outskirts Press, Inc.
http://www.outskirtspress.com

ISBN: 978-1-4787-0924-4

Outskirts Press and the "OP" logo are trademarks belonging to Outskirts Press, Inc.

PRINTED IN THE UNITED STATES OF AMERICA

I shot an arrow into the air,
It fell to earth, I knew not where;
For so swiftly it flew, the sight
Could not follow it in its flight.

I breathed a song into the air,
It fell to earth, I knew not where;
For, who has sight so keen and strong,
That it can follow the flight of song?

Long, long afterward, in an oak
I found the arrow, still unbroke;
And the song, from beginning to end,
I found again in the heart of a friend.

—*Henry Wadsworth Longfellow*

Table of Contents

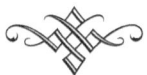

The Story

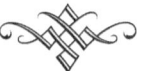

Once upon a time and long ago, there were two women who became friends. One was older and one was younger, but they were very much alike in personality. Both of them were smart and perceptive, liked music, were intrigued with the mysteries of the universe, loved God, and had a delightful sense of humor. The time they spent together was filled with laughter and storytelling. The older woman taught the younger woman many things, like what type of plants to put in her flower garden in order to have blooms from spring into fall, and how to attract different varieties of birds to her feeders. The younger woman liked to think that she taught the older woman a few things as well; things like daring to swim in the sea even if you couldn't swim, because the salt water would keep you afloat, and that sometimes having ice cream for dinner was just perfect. Yes, the two women together formed a perfect friendship, a union of souls, destined to last a long, long time.

Over the years their shared love of mission work took them more than once to Mississippi to help with the Hurricane Katrina recovery and to the Indian reservations in South

Dakota to work with their church. Painting and mucking out rooms was work made lighter with their constant joke-telling and laughter. Upon finding out how well-suited they were as travel companions they soon embarked on leisure trips together. Cruising down the Nile River gave way to never-ending practical jokes they played upon each other, teasing tales that gave way to gales of laughter when the ruse was discovered. The Greek Isles provided endless hours of thoughtful reflection together as well as much shopping and delightful Kodak moments. The two women sailed through the days of life together, each enriching the life of the other.

And then the dragon appeared. At first he watched and waited silently. Neither the older nor the younger woman was aware of his presence in the beginning. They were too busy living life. But the dragon was there nonetheless, watching and waiting for just the right time to devour the older woman. When he deemed the time ready, he sprang up with a mighty, fearful roar, and with fire spewing forth from his mouth, he began to chase the older woman. Caught totally unaware, the older woman ran for her life. The younger woman stayed by her side, hoping and praying that together they could avoid the dragon's relentless pursuit of the older woman. For many months, they were successful. The dragon seemed to retreat, and the two women cautiously hoped that the worst was over.

But the dragon had not forgotten nor given up his pursuit. He was silently building up his strength in order to devour the older woman more quickly at his next appearance, and when the dragon again deemed the time ready, he reared up, and with a mighty roar terrorized the older woman. She ran and ran, but still the dragon pursued her, ready to devour her if she slowed at all. Soon the older woman became tired. She felt the dragon gaining ground. The younger woman tried to encourage her to keep running, but even she could see that the older woman was losing momentum. She saw the fear in her beloved friend's eyes, and it made her afraid too.

The dragon was gaining ground. Any day now, he would overcome the older woman and devour her entirely. The older woman looked at the younger woman with sadness in her eyes, knowing that the time for farewells was close at hand. As they hugged for the last time, the younger woman knew she was losing someone very special, and she hated the dragon more than she ever hated anyone in her life. She cried and screamed at the dragon and prayed that someone would kill the dragon and save her beloved friend, but it was not to be.

That final day arrived. The older woman had no more strength left to run, so she sat quietly and waited for the dragon to claim her body. The younger woman sat with her, grieving and helpless to prevent the inevitable tragedy. As she held tightly onto the older woman's hands, the dragon pounced, devouring the older woman in an instant, and she was no more. The younger woman looked out at the world for the first time in many years without the older woman at her side, and it looked empty.

The dragon, unfilled by his recent act of carnage, immediately began looking anew for another unsuspecting victim to devour. All the people lived in fear of the dragon and his potential to appear suddenly in their own lives, because the dragon's name was Cancer.

Introduction

To everything there is a season…
a time to be born and a time to die.
Ecclesiastes 3:1-2

There is no greater grace and blessing than to be present at the birth of a baby. To watch this new human life take its first breath is simply a miracle to behold. It is difficult to imagine anyone denying the existence of a good and gracious God at this moment. I have had the opportunity to witness new life on multiple occasions; first, with my own three children, and then with my godchild, and finally with my first grandchild. These are holy moments that will be forever imprinted on my heart and soul.

Birth is also a moment filled with opportunity. The future is wide open for this new little life. Watching as the newborn grows and develops its own personality, with hopes and dreams of its own, reminds me of a saying I read years ago: *You hold your children's hand for a while but their hearts forever.* I don't know who authored that saying, but it is certainly a truism.

Eventually, if you've done your job well, they must become independent of you. The proverbial umbilical cord must be cut, so they can discover their God-inspired reason for being. Such is the cycle of life.

While you do have these little ones in your care, though, delight in them. Children teach adults things we have forgotten, things like how much fun rain puddles are or the joy of making a snow angel on newly fallen snow or seeing what pictures can be made out of cloud formations on a lazy summer afternoon. These are good things, wholesome and pure, that cause us to pause and ponder. Children, fresh from God, remember this. They are not jaded by life's experiences yet. Enjoy the children, for they feed our souls.

Then there is the other end of this spectrum we call life. We don't like it as much, and we make every attempt to ignore its eventuality. Death does not receive the same joyful acceptance that birth receives. Once we are incarnated, we tend to want to remain incarnated for better or for worse. We forget where we came from. As Christians, we know we belong to God and that He has prepared a place for us when we leave this earthly existence. Jesus tells us it is so in Matthew 14:2-3: *In my Father's house are many rooms. I go to prepare a place for you...* and yet the inevitable departure remains difficult for us. We are leaving our family and our friends. We may feel we have not accomplished all the things we wanted before we died. Our bucket list might not be all crossed off yet. We like it here, even if it's not the paradise promised to us. Earth's incarnation is a known commodity, versus the eternal glory our newborn self has long forgotten. Perhaps most daunting is that we make the departure from our physical body to our heavenly body by ourselves. None of our loved ones with skin still on are coming with us. It's like traveling to a foreign country alone. You may have read about it and felt confident about your journey, but there is still that little bit of trepidation when you actually set out. It usually doesn't fully go away until you set foot in the new land.

Walking with someone who is dying isn't exactly easy, either, for most of us for the same reasons. You are losing someone you love dearly. As Christians we believe they will be in a better place with all the glory promised to us in the Bible. It feels almost selfish to want them to remain here on earth with us, especially if they are suffering. It is a conundrum with no solution, and it causes us tremendous pain, both during the dying process and then afterwards, when we must go on with life without them.

There are many times when I have had some exciting news of some sort and have rushed to the phone only to remember that the person I am calling is no more. The pain lessens over time, but the person's absence is felt forever. I have railed at death and I have pleaded with God, but in the end, the human condition prevails. Death, of course, does not win ultimately; we know that, but knowing the theology behind death does not remove the physical grieving.

All that being said, there are some people who by their dying show us how to live. They allow us to make the walk into eternity alongside them, and they teach us how to die with dignity and grace. It is a blessing bestowed upon us unaware. Nonetheless, it is important for us to recognize this gift. To be allowed to be present with someone as he or she enters into eternal life is every bit the grace and blessing as being present for a birth. It is every bit as powerful. We fail to see the blessing, because consumed with our grief, the gift is veiled. Only as the grief subsides do we become aware of the blessings we are left with. It is up to us then to accept these blessings and be transformed by them or remain locked in our grief and miss the lesson.

I have chosen to accept the gift and let its blessing transform my soul. The journey has not been an easy one. I have spent myself in tears more than once. Grief has threatened to overwhelm me and has caused me to sink into despair on more than one occasion. I know in my heart of hearts that my dear friend is safe in the arms of God. I believe in His promise, but I still want her here. I want to call her on the phone. I want to have three- and four-hour dinners filled with laughter again. I want to travel to Bora Bora with her like we had planned. I feel abandoned and resentful that death has stolen one of my best friends from my life.

It is only now, almost three years after my friend Bea's death, that I can begin to see the gifts she has left me. It is only now that the raw grief of her passing has subsided somewhat that I can appreciate the blessing of being allowed to walk with her as the cancer slowly consumed her body. It is only now that I can also share these experiences with you.

How We Met

"Every time you smile at someone, it is an action of love,
a gift to that person, a beautiful thing."
—*Mother Teresa*

It might have been the twinkling blue eyes that first caught my attention. I never saw eyes that actually twinkled but Bea's did. They were a bright piercing blue color that reflected light like a prism, making everything about her sparkle and shine. Her movements were just as quick and full of an energy that belied her seventy-plus years. And she laughed. I don't mean every now and then she laughed. I mean Bea was a walking humor machine who loved nothing better than to play a prank or tell a joke. She was never malicious, though, and wouldn't hurt a fly if she could help it. It was just that she believed life was meant to be lived and not taken so seriously that you couldn't have a good laugh, even at your own expense sometimes.

We met at church, where we both happened to be serving on the parish council. I was attracted by her outgoing friendly personality that seemed to bubble up and out from somewhere deep within her soul. I have no clue what attracted her to me, although I suspect she would disagree with this statement. Being the only two women on the council at the time, we formed a sort of natural association. Little did either of us know at that time how intertwined our lives would become.

We were an interesting combination. Bea was a former nun who had parted ways from her order years earlier. I was a convert to the Catholic Church. There was a twenty-two-year age difference between us. Both of us had been married, and both of us had been divorced for many years. We shared a love of animals, books, music, talk—lots of it, and most important of all, our faith in God. We were both very adventurous and extremely independent, each of us spending many, many years in secular careers. While I had children of my own, Bea had acquired many throughout her forty-five years as a teacher. We both complimented and challenged each other with a kind of grace that exists between kindred spirits.

Bea was already retired when we met and had suffered the loss of her dear friend Jo three years earlier. Since then she had prayed for a friend who would be as compatible and close to her as Jo had been. I don't know if I was what she prayed for, but apparently I was what she got. She laughed when I said that to her, but she placed my photo on her shelf right next to Jo's photo and reminded me often how special that placement was. I returned the compliment by placing her photo among those of my children and grandchildren.

In those beginning years of our friendship, we began to share in each other's ventures. She became active in the vocations committee, spending many hours praying for vocations and finding ways to encourage others not only to pray for vocations, but also to consider a vocation with the church as well. Meanwhile, I began several ministries, including our church's

Red Hat group, dubbed the Holy Hatters. I founded the Holy Hatters and headed the group for one year, at which time Bea succeeded me as the queen mother.

During her tenure as queen mother, she arranged for the group to spend the night at the Marriott Hotel. We arrived to a prediction of a huge snowstorm that was to occur overnight. Never one to let a little snow get in the way of things, we played games—which included prizes, ate snacks, drank wine, and swam the night away. It was delightful to watch the snow gently falling outside as we swam in an eighty-degree pool. In the morning we had breakfast together and took pictures of the group dressed in our red and purple attire, blissfully unaware of how much snow had actually fallen during the night. Imagine our surprise when we headed out to find our cars buried under ten inches of snow! As we all cleared the snow off our cars, the only sound to be heard was Bea's laughter as she playfully lobbed snowballs at us, which we obligingly lobbed back at her. It was a perfectly delightful ending to a perfectly delightful weekend.

The Holy Hatters also had a white teddy bear with a red felt hat and purple boa, as our mascot. Our honorary bear sang "Girls Just Wanna Have Fun." This little bear, who resided with whoever was the current queen mother, accompanied us to our various events and to our annual meeting, dutifully singing at least once each time. It spent two years living with Queen Bea, a.k.a. Lady Painterly, perched atop her shelf and surrounded by Red Hat pictures and knickknacks. Today that bear sits on the top of my hutch, a silent but pleasant reminder of happier and more carefree times.

During our more serious times, Bea and I would spend hours exploring our spiritual interests together. Though conventional, conservative, and traditional in practice, we remained open-minded to other spiritualties and spent long hours discussing our thoughts. One book in particular captured our interest and was to become an important piece of our journey, although we didn't know it at the time. *The Sacred Contract* by Caroline Myss presented us with an interesting thought: what if we had our current life pre-planned by us, with the guidance of angels, in order to have a specific human experience, and all the people around us had agreed to accompany us on this journey, to fulfill their wish for a specific human experience as well as play a part in ours? What if? Think about it. It would certainly make forgiveness easier to do, on some level. It would also allow us to accept what comes our way in life, with the understanding that we chose to experience it in that particular way for our personal and spiritual growth. Although we never could reconcile this theory with our Catholic faith, it remained an intriguing *what if* that followed us through Bea's cancer journey, and it continues to bring me a measure of peace as I move on in life without her.

These long spiritual discussions took place in various venues; her home, my home, and any restaurant that would allow us to sit for three or four hours talking, and they led us to Noodles & Co. on more than one occasion. We ordered our food, took a back booth, and began to talk. Much of our opening dialogue centered on catching up on each other's activities while we ate. The conversation would then meander into discussing recent books or movies that almost always led us into the moral, ethical, or spiritual realm. Resurfacing from these discussions always caught us by surprise as we laughed at how much time had gone by. No topics were off-limits, and we each gave the other something to ponder when we parted ways again.

One topic that Bea brought up many times was her continued experience with certain smells that would appear out of nowhere, grab her attention, and then disappear just as quickly. Most of the time she claimed they were sweet floral smells, as if someone had been in that spot holding fragrant flowers. Although never able to identify the particular flower associated with the smell, she still knew it was floral, and being a master gardener, she certainly knew her flowers. Beyond that, she said the smells occurred at times when she needed comfort or assurance, and she believed that they were signs from family members or friends who had passed on or were gifts from the angels themselves. Many times these floral smells would occur during her prayer time, and they gave her much peace.

For the most part, even though I had my own unique spiritual experiences, I was slightly doubtful of her claim of smells. I wasn't sure smells could appear and then disappear just as quickly. My logical mind just couldn't wrap around that concept. I prayed for understanding, and one day I came upon an article that totally blew me away. The article was called "The Odor of Sanctity," and it described in detail what Bea had been sharing with me for years. I sent her the article by e-mail, and we had a wonderful discussion on the topic a few days later. After that, I was somewhat envious of her gift.

The beautiful ending to this is that sometime later, I too was blessed with a gift of floral smells, and had Bea not shared her experiences with me, I would not have understood this wonderful gift. At the time, my dad was dying of renal failure, and we had all gathered around for what we knew was imminent. Two of my daughters and I were standing around his bed when the entire area where he lay became filled with the most pungent, sweet-smelling floral scents. I stepped away from the bed, and the smell was not there, but when I returned to his bedside, the area was full of floral smells. As my daughters looked to me for clarity on what was happening, I simply said the angels were coming for him soon, and the floral smells were for us so we would know he was going home to heaven. The smells were meant to offer us comfort and strengthen our faith. Although I have never had another experience with the odor of sanctity, that one gift made all the difference.

Travels

"I've learned that goodbyes will always hurt; pictures will never replace having been there; memories good and bad will bring tears; and words can never replace feelings."
—*Unknown*

Ah, the joy of traveling to new places, discovering new treasures, and creating new memories. I used to tell my children that with every new adventure (or misadventure, at times) we were making a memory. They sometimes smiled and sometimes groaned, but today those long-ago experiences remain in their minds as memories of experiences we shared together, and that's the whole point.

I love to travel and have done so extensively in my lifetime, visiting more than a dozen countries in Europe, Asia, and Africa. I have traveled alone and I have traveled with groups of friends. I have to say that in spite of all its messiness, at times I agree with Louie Armstrong: "It's a Wonderful World."

By the time I met up with Bea, both of us had a lot of individual travel experience under our belts. Both of us had traveled abroad, and we had a plethora of stories and pictures to share with each other. Bea's favorite travel experience, and the one that intrigued me the most, was her excursion to Churchill, Canada, to see the migration of the polar bears. Her pictures were spectacular, and she had some wonderful tales to tell about the trip. Whenever she was asked about her travel experiences, this trip was always the first one she would tell about.

Bea was also a music teacher for forty-five years and an accomplished pianist. One of her most cherished memories as a teacher occurred in 1988. Bea spent three months that summer in Ichon, Korea, with the UNESCO program as a teacher in its English Summer School Program. Every picture taken during those three months had its own story, which she shared in such a way that you felt you had had the experience right alongside her. Bea infused each tale with such gusto, enthusiasm, and excitement that a person could sit and listen to her for hours.

My favorite trip has always been to the Holy Land. I have been there twice and would most certainly go there again. Despite the violence and clashes that erupt daily in Israel, there is something very special about walking on holy ground that transcends all of that chaos. Every time I look at my pictures of sunrise on the Sea of Galilee, I am instantly transported back there. The Gospel can never again be read and understood in the same way once you have walked in those very places described in the Bible. Bea had never traveled to the Holy Land, so I had the opportunity to share my pictures and experiences with her.

Another favorite trip of mine was to the Greek Isles. Both Bea and I had traveled there individually on previous occasions. In 2008, we had the good fortune to be able to travel there together. It turned out to be the last time we would ever travel together, since she was diagnosed with cancer shortly after we returned home. I look back at those pictures with both happiness and sadness now. They say hindsight is always 100%, and I guess that's true, but I would give anything to go back and relive that trip one more time.

For one thing, the Greek Isles are just plain stunningly beautiful. Sunsets are a kaleidoscope of colors bouncing off the white buildings. It would seem that God made the Greek Isles specifically for romantics and poets alike, although great scholars also claim a piece of that pie. It has all the beauty and history and drama that one could hope for. It was on the island of Patmos that St. John wrote the book of Revelation. I have visited the spot twice, both times coming away with new spiritual insights. The island of Rhodes contains a unique combination of both the old and the new, and then there is Santorini. I don't think I have ever seen a more beautiful spot on earth. Built high above the water, it explodes with a prism of color during the evening hours as the sun sets over the glistening sea. I have never seen anything quite like it, and it is quite intoxicating.

For another thing, Bea and I shared some of our most memorable laughs on that trip. First, our cabin aboard ship offered us a glimpse of how differently we arose in the morning. Bea was up talking and bustling about the minute she opened her eyes. I am too, after I've had some coffee. I like to ease into the day, so on our first morning aboard ship, you can imagine the scenario as she popped out of bed, threw open the curtains, and pulled down my bed sheets as she sang

some goofy song about rise and shine. Uh huh. We had a
nice conversation later that day about the do's and don'ts of
morning protocol. That story got told more than once and
still makes me chuckle.

Bea was not a swimmer, while I love to be in the water, so
in every port where we docked, my first mission was to find
a place to swim. Bea came along, mostly, I think, because she
was worried I'd drown in the sea. One day we docked in a tiny
port that had the most gorgeous beach. Since we were going
to be in this spot for a couple of days, I convinced her one
very hot afternoon to come and swim with me at the beach. It
was crowded, but we managed to find ourselves two reclining
chairs with attached umbrellas to shade us from the sun. Soon
we became a bit overheated and decided to head for the water.
I swam out to the ropes, delighted with the buoyancy of the
salt water. Bea, who could not swim a stroke, stayed near the
shore. Swimming back in to where she was sitting in the water,
I explained that this was the perfect time to swim, since the salt
water wouldn't let you sink. After much coaxing and cajoling,
I got her to come away from shore and experience the thrill of
swimming in the sea. After that she was a swimming fool! I no
longer had to coax her to go in the water when we reached a
new port. She was ready.

Back sitting in our umbrella-covered reclining beach chairs,
we decided to take a picture of each other for posterity. She
took my picture, and then I got up to take her picture. She
fussed over the seating, the placement of her towel, her hat, and
sunglasses. Everything had to be just right. Finally she got herself situated just right. Perched at the very end of her chair, she
posed for the picture. Just as I was about to snap the picture,
it happened. Bea had situated herself on the end of the long
reclining beach chair, which meant all the weight was on one

end, and just like that, at the moment of photography perfection, the whole thing collapsed and dumped Bea into the sand. She was mortified, and I was hysterical with laughter. So was the crowd around us. She was a good sport about the whole event and laughed right along with us, but she wasn't game to try for another picture. Because I was laughing so hard, I missed the best Kodak moment of the trip. The memory still makes me laugh out loud today, and I know Bea is giggling with me from up in heaven.

Our first mission trip together occurred in April 2006; eight months after Hurricane Katrina decimated the Gulf Coast. For all the media attention given to New Orleans, most people forget the eye of the hurricane passed directly over the Waveland / Bay St. Louis, Mississippi area. This area was chosen by our archdiocese for relief work. Bea and I made that initial trip in April to survey the area and meet the people we would be working with before returning home to help churches prepare to send work groups down. The leader of the archdiocesan project, dubbed Rebuilding Lives Restoring Hope, was Fr. Paul Esser. He had previously made the trip to Mississippi in January, to meet with the pastors in the area and discover where we could be of most help.

The pastor of Our Lady of the Gulf Parish graciously allowed us to stay in one of the FEMA trailers located on church grounds. Neither of us had ever been to a disaster area, and the sights were overwhelming. Driving in our rented car from the airport, we were abruptly stopped by the outage of the bridge connecting Pass Christian to Bay St. Louis, which meant a lengthy drive around with sketchy directions because all visible landmarks to guide us were gone: "Turn right at the huge rubbish pile about one mile down the road and then left at the school and follow the road until you come to a wall with a huge

X on it." You get the picture. People were very kind and friendly to us, in spite of the horrendous thing that had just happened to them, and we arrived in less time than we imagined.

Arrived where would have been the better question. Eight months after Katrina came ashore, the wreckage remained unchanged. There were signs of hope, though: one fast food restaurant was open, and one breakfast restaurant, one grocery/supply store, and one gas station. Tent cities for volunteers from around the country were located in Waveland and Kiln. FEMA trailers filled every vacant piece of land for survivors who chose to live in them and restore their homes or rebuild, as the case may be. Mucking out houses, hauling out debris, and waiting in long lines for everything became the MO of volunteers and locals alike.

For Bea and me, it was baptism by fire. By day we worked wherever we were needed, and by night we ate, talked, and spent time with the other volunteers or the many local people who invited us to share a meal with them. We sat by bonfires after eating wonderful shrimp boils, and we sat in FEMA trailers listening to stories of survival. The experience changed us. Mission work starts out as helping others, but it almost invariably ends up giving back so much more. It is a truism that anyone, on any level of involvement, will attest to.

One thing that stood out during that week in Mississippi was the complete lack of wild animal life. There were no birds, no squirrels, and no life forms other than human that we could see. We were wrong. It was springtime, and springtime in the South brought the arrival of the no-see-ums. These are tiny little gnats that, well, you can't see. They also had hard shells for bodies that made it darn near impossible to kill them when they bit you. Even if you couldn't see these nasty little critters, you could sure feel their bites.

Everyone seemed to have a different theory on what people could spray on themselves to keep the no-see-ums away. Bea and I were northerners. We don't have so-see-ums where we live, much less have any type of biting bugs in the early spring, so it never entered our minds to bring any type of bug spray with us. The one store that was open was continually out of stock, obviously having sold out to people who had done a better job at educating themselves about their surroundings. We toughed it out and tried to stay covered up as much as possible, which was no easy task, with temperatures in the eighties and very humid. Somehow we still managed to find the humor in our predicament and made up silly songs and poems about these tiny carnivorous flying beasts. They got the last laugh, though, because after we returned home, we both had to go to the doctor for steroid shots to combat the allergic reaction our bodies were experiencing as a result of the many bites we each had on our ankles, arms, and legs. Bea suffered more than I did from the no-see-ums, because some of her bites became infected, and she had to be treated for infection, too. Of course she made up comical theories as to why she was a more popular host for the insects, and because of her wonderful ability to turn any situation into an *I Love Lucy* parody, today I can look back on that memory and chuckle instead of shudder.

Our last mission trip together took us to a church located on an Indian Reservation in Marty, South Dakota. Bea and another member of our church had spearheaded this twinning project, and our volunteer church work groups had already made a few trips there. This particular trip was in July 2007, and it was quite hot. Our large group split up into smaller groups and headed out each day to do various work projects on the reservation. Our lodging was either in a hotel or in cabins next to a lake at a nearby campground. Bea, another friend, and I stayed in a cabin with a beautiful view of the water.

If you have ever camped, then you know that camping cabins do not come equipped with their own bathroom amenities. For those concerns, you usually need to leave your cabin and walk some distance to the communal facilities. This isn't an issue, unless it happens to be the middle of the night and you need to use those facilities. A word of advice: people who have these needs regularly should stay in a hotel. I'm just saying.

Anyway, as happened with some regularity, each of us usually had to make the long, dark trek to the bathroom at some point during the night. This hike was particularly unnerving to me, because I am afraid of the dark. I can travel around the world and work with dying people in the slums of Calcutta, but a walk to the bathroom in the middle of the night in a campground full of people terrifies me. Go figure, but there it is. I tried very hard not to drink anything for hours before bedtime, to avoid my nemesis. Sometimes it worked, and sometimes I just had to face my demons.

Bea, on the other hand, had no such idiosyncrasy. "When you gotta go, you gotta go" was her motto. One night she got up and groggily left to fulfill that motto. Unfortunately, the shoes she put on had smooth, slippery bottoms, and the stairs outside were wet with dew. The combination resulted in a nasty fall that left her entire leg, from hip to knee, black and blue. She rested for one day and then insisted on getting back to work with the rest of us. It was hot, she was hurt, and we all watched her like a hawk, but she was a trooper and painted along with the rest of us for the next two days.

She was seventy-five years old on this trip, and she constantly amazed me. It wasn't just her stamina and vitality. It was more than that. Bea breathed life into everything. She made everything, every experience more fun. It was more than that too. She had the rare ability to make you understand that you were so much more than you gave yourself credit for too.

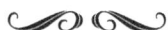

The Journey Changes

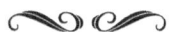

The Diagnosis

You can close your eyes to the things you do not want to see, but you cannot close your heart to the things you do not want to feel.

—*Unknown*

Bea left for her long-awaited cruise to the Virgin Islands with a church friend in January 2009. She wasn't feeling well, but attributed it to her recurring gastrointestinal problems. She had some longstanding medical problems with liver cysts and reflux that kept her in touch with her doctors on a regular basis for monitoring, so she brought her meds with her and sailed off without a second thought. She was gone for two weeks. I was busy working, and the time passed quickly in her absence.

I was eager to see and hear all about her trip upon her return, but she informed me that she had gotten very sick on the last day of her trip and had made a doctor appointment as soon as she had arrived home. She couldn't keep food down and was afraid she had some type of intestinal bug. Not wanting to infect anyone else, she promised to keep me informed. I heard nothing more until I received her call from the hospital. I was at work, and she told me they wanted to do some tests and also give her some IV fluids. Her inability to keep foods down had left her dehydrated. She didn't sound any more worried than expected at this point, and I said I would visit when I got out of work.

"My long awaited cruise to the Virgin Islands in January changed everything almost in an instant. The last two days of the trip, I knew there was something wrong. I wasn't feeling all that great when I started out, but figured it was my GERD problem kicking up and knew how to deal with it.

January 19, I returned home, and on the twentieth, called the doctor and got an appointment right away. I was treated for either GERD or the flu. That week I spent mostly in the ER, as nothing stayed down and I was getting dehydrated. The following Monday, I had an endoscope and found there was a blockage in the duodenum. I was admitted to the hospital that day, hoping to have the blockage shrink...biopsy showed there was no cancer. All scopes, MRI, CAT scans showed nothing out of the ordinary...no cancer...everything was stable. From January 27 to February 2 I lived on IVs. On February 2, the doctor performed surgery to have a new opening for the stomach, so I could eat. Upon opening me up, he discovered I had inoperable cancer called periampullary cholangio pancreatic carcinoma."

Visiting Bea during those days before the surgery turned into a roller coaster ride of emotions for us. With every test we held our breath and waited for the results, praying for a benign result, and every test *did* come back benign. For some reason, the tumor was tucked away in her abdomen in an area untouched by the scopes. It was only when they opened her up that they discovered the massive cancerous tumor intertwined with many blood vessels and organs, which made it impossible to remove.

In the days preceding her surgery, Bea was her usual jovial self, for the most part. Every benign test result gave way to sighs of relief. It was as if the future had been given back, and this was just a nasty scare. To help pass the time, I brought Bea some colored pencils and drawing paper. I figured it would give her something to do and allow the creative life juices to flow again. She created some wonderful floral pictures during the week she was in the hospital prior to surgery. The pictures decorated the bulletin board in her room and helped make it seem less clinical.

We had some long spiritual talks during this time as we pondered the meaning of what was occurring. We referred to *The Sacred Contract* and joked that if it were true, why would we pick this path? We talked about the "what ifs" that could manifest from this experience. We were encouraged by the good test results so far, but were apprehensive of the blockage that was still inside of her. While we spoke of many things, the unspoken words of fear were expressed solely between our eyes when we looked at each other. It was like if we didn't give words to those fears, then they would not manifest themselves in reality. We went on like that until the day of surgery.

"I remember the doctor bending over me while I was in the morphine state telling me I had cancer, but there was hope for treatment, but not a cure. The cancer was entwined in too many vessels, and I would have bled to death while the doctor was trying to unwrap all of it. My response was, 'my one-way ticket to heaven,' and then I fell asleep. Somehow I knew this information for a long time. My sixth sense kept telling me I had cancer, but I'd dismiss it, thinking you are what your thought life is, so be gone, negative thoughts…and that was all during the summer and fall of 2008.

I was told the cancer was there anywhere from three to four years already, and it was slow growing, which made treatment and recovery more positive to deal with.

I was heavily dosed in morphine; when alert I could barely pray, but I remember just letting myself bask in His loving presence. What sustained me up to this point was centering prayer. Though I fell asleep many times, because of the morphine, I knew I was being held in His arms. Looking back, there was only one set of footprints in the sand as He was carrying me, protecting me, giving me strength."

I received the phone call at work. My daughter was a surgical nurse at the time of Bea's surgery. Bea had requested my daughter be her nurse for surgery and had also given my daughter permission to call me with the results of the surgery. Because all of the tests had come back favorable, I was not overly concerned regarding diagnosis, when I answered the call. At the time I just wanted to make sure Bea had made it through surgery okay. She was seventy-eight years old, and this was a huge surgery she was undergoing.

All I remember hearing from that call were the words *pancreatic cancer*. My entire being went numb as the shock slammed into me: pancreatic cancer, the worst kind, and the most deadly. It was not the first time this diagnosis had touched my life. My mother died in 1997 of pancreatic cancer. She endured surgery, radiation, and chemotherapy for four and a half years before succumbing to the disease. It was one of the worst times of my life, and I was about to experience it all over again.

Certainly when a diagnosis like this strikes, the focus is on the patient, as well it should be. After all, the person with the disease now has to focus on treatment and survival, and those around must step up and be a support system. But the impact a diagnosis of cancer has on those who will make the "walk with" brings its own struggle. That struggle is one of helplessness to change anything that is happening. The emotions are different from the emotions born of survival, but they are there ,and they can be very conflicting.

I felt very much like a two-year-old having an internal temper tantrum. I did not want to experience the march through pancreatic cancer again—ever. I did not want to lose my friend. I did not want to watch the disease ravage her as it did my mother. I did not want to hope and pray the disease was eradicated with every remission. I did not want to feel the pain and fear related to every relapse. I also felt guilty for feeling this way, while my friend was fighting for her life. Unlike my walk with my mother, this time I knew I had to find a support system.

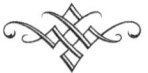

The Journey

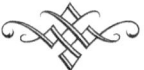

"Those who don't know how to weep with their whole heart don't know how to laugh either."
—*Golda Meir*

Bea came home from the hospital on February 12, 2009. She still had a drainage tube in her side and staples holding her incision closed. The doctor had assured her that she would be treated aggressively. He made it clear he could not promise her days, weeks, months, or years, but he did promise he would do everything to enhance the quality of her life.

"My treatment of Gemzar began on March 5, [and I went] every week until May, and then I went three weeks in a row with one week off until September. I had four weeks off, and then began five and a half weeks of radiation, Monday through Friday, while carrying a chemo pack on my hip called 5FU with an infusion being delivered every eight minutes, twenty-four/seven, Monday through Friday. I had the weekend off. This [routine] ended October 21, 2009.

As of the writing of this account, I have lab work to be done twice a month yet, and the doctor on December 7. At that time, future scans and tests will be appointed, and [I] will probably know by the end of December whether or not all the treatments did their work."

It was during her months of treatments that I encouraged her to keep a journal. I have kept a journal for years now, and I find it to be both helpful and insightful. I thought it would do the same for Bea. At the time, neither of us had any thoughts of making her journal public. That discussion would take place during her final week of life as she lay in the hospital. It was then that we talked about sharing her cancer journey. Knowing at that point she would not be here to see the project to fruition, she wrote and signed her permission for me to use her journal to tell this story.

Home again! Looking back, I see how things have worked from February 12 until the present. Reading was impossible for the first few months; neither eyes nor attention would focus. All I could manage was getting out of bed with rubber knees and a sickening feeling all over my body. I made it getting my coffee, looking over the paper—my favorite was the comics, as I had a chance to laugh. This also carried over to my computer, as friends sent me jokes and such to laugh about. My computer, by the way, was my connection to the outside with friends and family, as was the phone.

I was able to make a breakfast, but many times no strength to clean up…the lounge chair became my safe landing place, until I could gather more energy to finish the job. I complained to the doctor that it took me three days to finish a job, whereas I used to do three days' worth in one day. His response was, "You are recuperating from surgery and will soon recuperate from poison that will be injected into your body—chemo infusions—be patient." Patience is the least of my virtues.

Once I got the all-clear to drive again, I decided my first venture would be to the grocery store. By the time I got there, my legs and arms were feeling like they belonged to a puppet, and the puppeteer didn't know how to work the ropes, so there I stood, holding onto the grocery cart, wondering if I should just go home or give it a try. All I could do that day were two aisles, and went home, left the bags in the car, and found my lounge chair. The next day I did another portion of the shopping, and the same the following day. It took three days to finish, but I did it, and that was encouraging… talk about patience and endurance! I cried.

The lounge chair was my safe place where I spent many hours, gradually centering in prayer and, of course, learning a deeper way of praying to the Father. Listening brought up in my inner being things from the time I was a child to now. I reflected how I had been gifted in so many ways…my parents, grandparents, family, friends, learning to be a dancer, taking music lessons, growing up among people who loved me and inspired me, being a successful teacher for forty-five years, and becoming an artist after retiring and being in many juried shows and galleries.

Also, unresolved conflicts came up, and I was given time to reflect and resolve, make willful intentions to forgive what was real or imaginary on my part, and send healing thoughts to those I offended. Looking at all this, I think it right to say that suffering and illnesses are a gift if taken in the right spirit…this surely has been my gift. Oh, my, there were so many gifts I have been given; it was overwhelming, and here I was stuck with cancer right at the peak of my "good life." Yes, I cried many times. I gave myself permission to do that, as it was a good cleansing of mind and heart.

Then there was March 5, my first chemo infusion. As I sat in the chair getting the chemo, the whole reality kicked in. Tears came, and I tried not to cry out loud. Looking around me, I saw others going through the same thing. Some were laughing while visiting with family; others were reading, and some had their eyes closed. I leaned back, closed my eyes, and put myself in His presence.

During all this time, my favorite prayer was and still is, "If my presence on earth is to continue your creation, bless me with healing of both mind and body. If my presence is no longer needed to carry out your creation, give me healing of mind and body to say with an open heart, Thy will be done." I'd add, "Dear God, it's hard to say 'Thy will be done,' but know I am saying it with my will...that's the best I can do right now, as I sure can't feel it!"

Living with the what if questions, the uncertainty of my future...I am gradually beginning to pray and ponder about that. Sometimes I can almost feel a voice (I don't hear voices, let me tell you) that inner voice that I feel responds when I ask God the Father the question, "Will I ever get cured?" and then that voice comes back, "Be patient; everything will work out in My good time." That's what sustains me in periods of doubt, anxiety, and fear. Of course I pray for a miracle. I tell the Father that I believe He is all powerful, all good, all merciful, and to look at me in my misery and grant me a cure.

This cancer journey did not all take place in a week, but many, many days. It all started in January, the new phase of my life wherein we are all destined to spend some time suffering long periods of illnesses before we can leave this world. You see, we all know about these things; we've read about them, but to be thrown into a situation where one really has to live it is something else. I guess that's what wisdom is, knowing versus living a truth.

Let me just go back to the suffering part and glean some insights gotten through many homilies and readings. Suffering is everyone's lot. What it does is give you a chance to have a sabbatical with the Lord. Yes, it takes you out of the mainstream of worldly things, so you can reflect and get closer to where God wants you to be in the first place. I figured I had gotten so involved in things that God was getting shortchanged. I have had time to center on what's important, and I hope I have grown a little bit closer and wiser spiritually. I have found ways and more meaning to "fill up what is wanting in the sufferings of Christ," as St. Paul says. That was always a mystery to me, but I think I am getting a little better understanding of that. Faith. That is what has gotten me this far. Another gift.

Now for the miracles and cures; there are miracles all around us every day, every minute. The sunrise; the sunset; the rain to water the earth; the sun to give life; fruits, vegetables, and flowers grow to give nourishment for body and soul; medicines; and the list goes on and on. But the miracles for cures lie in the gifts given to the doctors who have the ability to diagnose and treat our illnesses. They can extend a person's life until it is the person's time to leave this world. They cannot make a cure happen instantly; only God can do that. Doctors can cure only for a time, and that differs from patient to patient. My hope and desire is that I'll be around for a long time. I'm a realist; my type of cancer is not curable, and that's a fact. I will rejoice in the time I am free of cancer but be ready, with God's help, to meet whatever comes next and make decisions at that time. I know one day it will pop up again; when and where, I don't know. What is important is to live in the now and see every day as a gift and do what needs to be done just for today.

Resilience. Never gave that word much thought, but I wondered how I got it. Children learn what they see. My parents went through some tough times when I was just a child. Dad almost died when I was seven years old. As I look back, he never complained during his recuperation. He took care of his family despite the fact that he wore a tracheal tube for many years, because of his throat paralysis, and he found a way to make us laugh and enjoy each other. He was given the wrong type of blood during an appendectomy operation, and a blood clot formed at the base of his skull, paralyzing his breathing.

Perhaps it was during this part of my growing up that I learned how to pray with faith. The whole family went to church every Tuesday and Friday night to pray that my dad would be healed. We were told that he would never be without a tracheal tube, never smell or taste food again, never go in a boat for fear of falling in the water, and never go swimming. Talk about resilience! We prayed for twelve years, and finally my dad's sense of smell and taste returned. The tracheal tube fell out one morning, and he discovered he was able to breathe on his own again, so they closed the opening in his throat for good.

Mother almost died when I was around twelve years old, and like Dad, she never complained. She bounced back and took care of the family. Although their health was compromised the rest of their lives after those setbacks, Dad lived to be seventy-eight, and mother passed away at the age of eighty-six.

Someone asked me halfway into my journey of cancer if what I was saying about how I was handling my illness is what I really meant, or if I was just parroting someone else's thoughts. That sure made me stop and think, but I have to admit, my handling of this illness could be found only in the one and only source of strength: God, my heavenly Father. How does one survive it alone?

God's Proof of His Presence

My friend Jo and I took care of our aging parents until gradually, one by one, they passed away. I ranted once again when my father passed away with an aneurism on July 24, 1984. I talked to my God, asking him why I never got to say goodbye to him. I even remember standing by my dad's grave, angry that he went so fast. I was obsessed constantly with "What is heaven, and what happens when you get there; what is my dad doing, and is he all right?" In August I had a dream, one of those that come in the early morning hours, just before I awakened. My dad stood next to my bed with his hand on my shoulder and said, "Everything is okay, Tootie,"

Only he called me that nickname. I knew it was him, as I could smell his flannel work shirt. It had the smell of factory oil. I knew for sure God had sent him to comfort me.

Mother passed away December 14, 1996. She broke her hip in June, and while she was in rehab, it was discovered she had pancreatic cancer, along with dementia. I watched her body shrink from the illness, and she gradually went into a coma. I sat for hours at her bedside, praying for her release from suffering. I told her many times I loved her. About a week after her funeral, she appeared in my dream as being very healthy, wearing her favorite clothes, and even had put on weight. She smiled at me as she walked away waving. Again, God let me know she was okay.

You would have thought after I was angry at the loss of my dear parents, God would have given up on me. I sure did have a mixture of being angry, sad, lost, and the whole ball of wax, even too exhausted at times to pray. If I prayed, it seemed like I was in a fog a lot of the time. Without my parents, I was alone, the next generation to be on the fast track to eternity, I thought. Mass and praying brought me through. I busied myself with a newfound outlet, art.

In December 1997, my friend Jo and I went to Florida for the winter. Returning home in March 1998, Jo began having problems that the doctors could not pinpoint. It wasn't until February 1999 that she was diagnosed with pancreatic cancer and lived only until April 8.

This was the ultimate blow. She was more my sister than a friend, and now I was really alone. We prayed together and had many spiritual talks, during which time we made a pact that I would take care of her until she died. I promised her that I would tell her, when the time came, to grab His hand and run like a deer. I made her promise she would send help when I was at my lowest and keep taking care of me.

I remember one day I was again so angry at the loss that I was crying and screaming at the same time, stamping my feet, hitting anything that wouldn't break (I wasn't so far off to destroy anything). I felt the need to get the anger out of my system. My poor dogs even hid. This feeling of despondency stayed with me all day, and when I went to bed, I prayed for relief and then reminded Jo she promised to help me out when I got to a low point. My crying stopped. I felt relaxed and fell asleep.

My angel dream then came. I was being pressed on both sides by two tall beings in white, but I couldn't see their faces or feet. They kept pressing me very hard, trying to turn me away from the blackness I was looking at. Like a wiener in a bun, I slipped around and saw the most beautiful circle of light (I tried many times to reproduce it in watercolor, but it was never anything like I saw) and I heard a voice saying, "Be at peace; it was God's will." I woke up. It was 3:00 a.m. I sat up in bed and was aware of a smell like washed linen that had been on the clothesline on a windy spring day. I sat up in bed, and for the longest time, the odor stayed and then floated away. I lay back on the pillow and fell into a deep sleep. When I woke up, I had the most wonderful feeling of peace. Never again did I feel despondent, but I did go through the normal grieving process. Once again God sent a sign of His presence by way of an angel.

Ever since then, whenever I have an irresolvable problem or am in a situation where I need comforting or help, I will experience for a minute or two a scent that is indefinable. This will happen in the early waking hours or during centering prayer. I welcome it and thank it, wondering if it is an angel, a spirit guide, or God Himself. Whoever it is, I know God sent the gift. How blessed I am to have received this gift! I guess my friend Jo is keeping her end of the promise to take care of me.

November 2, 2009

Yesterday we celebrated All Saints, and today, the departed saints (and my birthday). As I sit here looking out at my garden, this whole theme plays out the mystery every year: Life, death, and resurrection; a barren plot of earth where tiny seeds are dormant until the warm sun of spring nudges them to awaken; the summer months when we watch as the seedlings mature into a beautiful garden, lush, green, and colorful. As the warmth of the sun grows less and less with the coming fall, we see plants get frail and die, with only the hardy ones withstanding the first frost and continuing blooming into the late fall. Finally the death blow comes with a heavy freeze, and the garden becomes barren once more.

That's life. I am in the fall of my years, and I like to think I am one of the hardy plants. God is very near and talks to us through nature, just like my garden, all to keep us aware. I never looked at my garden that way before, but it sure keeps me grounded...no pun intended, either!

One other thing that has made this birthday different is I felt with each greeting from my friends that they might be thinking this could be my last. One of the women at church even touched my arm with a sad, knowing look. I do not want that kind of sympathy or thoughts interfering with my joy of each day, darn anyway! I plan to be around next year, just to prove God has his own plans for me...sure wish I knew what they were.

I found an old book I read long ago called The Loving Search for God *by W. Meninger. I did a lot of underlining in that book and am amazed those thoughts are still thoughts that guide me. A hard one is "Love begins when nothing is expected in return." If only that thought would be there when disturbing incidents occur, rather than hours or days later. A lot gets lost in the mayhem of daily life... a fault of our human condition...it seems I have a lot of that lately.*

November 11, 2009

One more crisis gone by…my liver is enlarged on my CAT scan. The results showed nothing to worry about, but I am concerned, as the last scan was inconclusive, and I wonder if this latest one falls into that category too. I've got to wait for the PET scan in December for a true picture. All this waiting is my hell on earth… will the PET scan show I still have cancer? Has it spread? Will I be put on palliative care? It does keep my eyes and attention on what is most important, staying connected to my God, who gives me strength and endurance.

All I know is this cancer will get me one of these days, and I want to be ready to pass over in peace. I steel myself for this coming event in my life. I hate thinking of being dependent in my last days. I don't want to be a burden to others. We all must suffer before we die; I know this; it is part of making up what is wanting in the suffering of Christ. That thought is such a mystery. I know and can feel it but cannot put it in words just yet. The meaning of putting on Christ is beginning to take on new meaning for me. I have resolved to use each day as that gift given to me, make the best of what comes, and live like I will live forever…to laugh, find joy in people around me, do ordinary things of daily life, and be at peace within and without.

I continue to survive and thrive each day, which is a gift in itself. Cancer changes one's perception of life. My control of things has changed. Making long-range plans is out of the picture. I have no control over my energy levels, my waiting for test results, managing my bouts of nausea, or feelings of anxiousness. One thing for sure: cancer cannot invade my soul or steal my eternal life or conquer my spirit. I can take command of my destiny, never be depressed over things that may never happen, be positive, hopeful at all times….I can do all things in Him, who strengthens me.

December 15, 2009 - Advent

Much has happened since November's CAT scan. I had the PET scan, and the cancer is still there on the pancreas, though diminished in size from the first and second scans. There is a possibility that it is residue from the radiation. The cancer has not spread as of this date. Another scan is scheduled for the week of February 8, and final results February 18. It is a "wait and see" if it grows or spreads. Other alternative treatments are in the wings, if that be the case.

This whole year, you might say, has been an Advent for me… waiting—seeking the light— chasing the monsters of worry out of my mind—WAITING…waiting…waiting…WAITING—and will continue that way, always waiting for test results to see where this cancer is going. This is my phase two, no treatments, but being monitored. Phase three will be treatment, if necessary, and if the cancer is untreatable, then on to palliative care. My quality of life right now is great. Today is December 15 and going strong.

My friend sent me some thoughts about time…reflecting on it. I was given the gift of life, and for seventy-nine years have been living in time, each day climbing closer to eternity. Jesus was born into time. He, the creator of time, became the servant of us all. Now, how am I living in this time to be the servant? There must be a reason I am still here. I cannot wallow in sadness, do or say anything that will make my friends and family overly concerned about my condition, and must never allow myself to live in emptiness. I have handed myself over to Him to lead me and use me, so I can say with an open heart, "Your will be done."

Monsters: spooky thoughts of "what if" keep crowding my mind. It is a struggle at times not to think about them, yet they are there, no matter how hard I try not to think about the "what ifs." Thoughts are only spooky when they are not seen—rationalized—the unknown is the spooky scary part of thoughts. Friends can give skin to the uncertainties, the spooks that crowd one's life, but it is not easy to unburden oneself. Solution? I let myself cry and complain to God when needed. I appreciate the listening ears of friends, but in the end, God is the one to disperse those monsters of what ifs.

Waiting: my patience has been strung out. I realize I have lost control of so many aspects of my life this year. This is the final preparation of my journey, a complete surrender. May I have the strength to allow this to happen with patience, forgiveness, love, and serving Him.

December 20, 2009

"Compassionate love showered on wounded spirits lights love's fire within." These words were taken from a quote on a card given to me by my friends Sisters Alice and Evelyn. To ponder that thought is difficult, but what it means to me is to take up my cross and follow Him. In my case, waiting has now become a time of preparation for that final passage, like the seeds in the pine cone that come to life—rebirthing—only when heated in a forest fire. Deep inside me are those seeds being carried as they rub raw sometimes, this disease of cancer, which at the same time allows me to walk with God, to take up my cross.

What can it teach me? Patience, tenderness, thoughtfulness, compassion, love, and forgiveness; the nuisance of being out of control, frustrated at times, and fearful of the future; continued fear of the next test results; patience, trust, and resignation.

I have to retreat into my own darkness to find the light, to understand the "why," to live by faith and hope. Whatever the outcome of my disease, I know He will keep me turned to the light and chase away the monsters of fear and what-ifs.

Perhaps I should be grateful that I have this disease and have time to walk through the fire of purification. If I had died instantly in an accident or suffered a stroke and lost the ability to think, talk, or respond, I would never have had this chance. What I have is golden, a gift, strange as it may sound. I can be an eternal storm against God with floods of petitions trying to change Him who calmed the sea, or I can surrender to God with an inner shift to adapt myself to God's own ebb and flow. That's the best part of waking up and seeing the Light, giving over my control of things that can't be changed. Thy will be done.

January 5, 2010

What a holiday this has been! Christmas Eve afternoon, I was in a car accident. No injuries, but again a reminder that life is unpredictable. One minute here, and the next you could be gone. I am still here. I had no real family to celebrate with, but I was embraced by many friends, the presence of God in my life through His people.

The meditation of January 4 said, "Life is an invitation to come and see where He is for us." As I move out of the stage of treatment and into the stage of wait-and-see, I realize I must stay in that place with patience, using it to grow spiritually. A test on January 18 and one on February 18; it is so difficult to wait for results. My whole life seems suspended, and every little twinge of pain makes me wonder if the cancer is growing out of control. The only thing that keeps me balanced is knowing He is beside me. I see this again in the friends I have who personify Him in the flesh.

January 8, 2010

I think of all the blessings I have been given throughout all my life. How can I share these blessings, especially now that I am not out among people as much as I had been? Being at peace with the situation I am in, give a smile to even those I don't know, gentleness, forgiveness, a sense of peace; all I know is I am still alive, which means my presence on earth is still needed to show His presence to others; that's my sharing in His creation. Lord, if you want you can make me clean…heal me.

January 11, 2010

"Come with me, and I will make you fishers of men," simple men who became leaders for His kingdom. There is nothing we do in this life—teacher, artist, friend, parent, family member, the list goes on—for building up of His kingdom. We were given gifts to become gifts to the world. How awesome a thought! Too bad it took me all these years to have it finally sink in. How much time I have left to actually live in the wisdom of that thought is unknown. All I know today is now, all the more reason to live in His presence, so I don't screw it all up! It gives true meaning to the phrase, "Lord, make me an instrument of your peace."

January 17, 2010

Today's Gospel retells the story of Cana and Mary's telling the servants to "do whatever He tells you to do." What needs to be done in my life here and now? I have put off volunteering, for fear I will not be around to finish the job. Who really is assured of that anyway? My job is to overcome that thought and do it anyway. I will volunteer to be a driver for a person undergoing chemo treatment who has no transportation. I intend to make the call Tuesday, after my endoscope is out of the way.

Let Him be in the driver's seat…take the wheel of what is to be.

February 16, 2010

A whole month has passed, and things sure went down the tube for me. From January 18 to February 7-8-9-10-11, it's been nothing but struggle. I entered the hospital on February 7 and came home on the eleventh, diagnosed with sepsis, a bad infection.

I was called on Sunday morning to report to the ER as an inpatient for antibiotic IV. While I was there, tests showed I had problems in the kidney and liver. My skin turned yellow. I had more tests and finally had a stent inserted into the liver to drain the bile. This procedure will be completed on the twenty-fourth of this month. Coming home was good, but very hard. As I am writing this, I am feeling very weak. Eating has been a problem, because of the lack of bile to break down the food—enzymes, they tell me.

I feel like this last episode is the beginning of the downward slip to the end of my cancer journey.

While in the hospital, I had a vision of two Order priests standing at the door of my room. They were dressed in an Order's black habit something like the Redemptorist Order. One had a white beard. I asked them what was going to happen, and they only smiled and left.

Several times while in my home, I felt many entities sitting in my living room, so I figured it was a sign that I have many spirit guides helping me through all this pain. The presence of God depends on the presence of God within us. I saw a video of the miracles of the Eucharist. I must say I have never doubted the true presence.

Am I discouraged? No. Sad? No. Fearful? A bit, yes. Can I cope? Yes, with the help of God and my angels, both in the flesh and the spirit.

It doesn't look like I will be volunteering just yet, as I have another procedure on the twenty-fourth.

April 3, 2010 - Holy Saturday

This Holy Week has been very different. I suffered along with the liturgy, I think, as I kept offering my inconveniences and pain. I must say I have gone through a change in many areas. I have lost quite a bit of weight now, and food is difficult to keep down.

I feel myself fading away and am sure I am on my last leg of the journey. It's funny how the taste of food, once so delectable, has become a source of pain and a chore. Is this what they call the beginning of detachment? Another thing, I am envious of those people who are able to get up and do things, when I have to sit around. Detachment?

Thank God for all my angel friends who shop for me, make me meals, do things I can no longer do…detachment…a preparation for the final departure. I still have a lot to shake off before then, I think. Funny, one never thinks about this when they are well. Dealing with this disease of cancer changes one's perspective of things. It's like watching your life gradually come to a stop in slow motion.

The last six weeks have been long and hard. I was in and out of the hospital for five days at a time, following a week in the nursing home, all of which took the starch right out of me. I finally came home and gradually got my walking legs back, but the food problem has gotten worse. All my strength now comes from centering prayer. God is my strength; I know for sure I could not do this on my own.

I am determined not to go to the ER this weekend, even though I have not been able to keep food down as I should. I will wait until Monday, when I go for my chemo, and get checked out with the doctor. Of course what is on my mind most is what the end will be and when it will come. I do not fear death. I just don't want it to linger, as that situation is very hard on those who are close and dear to me.

My Reiki practitioner told me she was aware of crowds of angels in my house. They said I should ask for what I want, and I keep telling them, "A remission of this cancer and return of my appetite and healing of my digestive system," but I guess that's not in my contract, and I must be true to my convictions. My work, my purpose on earth, is coming to a close, and with an open heart, I must say, "Not my will but Thy will be done."

Of course the doctor has not officially declared that I am nearing the last part of this journey, but I can feel it and am preparing myself.

Tomorrow is Easter Sunday, and I so hoped to go to Mass, but right now think I won't be able to make it.

All of 2009 was a roller coaster ride for me—physically, emotionally and mentally—beginning with Bea's surgery in early 2009. My dad's health was beginning to fail. He was ninety-one years old and had been in a nursing home since the previous summer. Age and illness were beginning to take a toll on his system, and he was spending more and more time in the hospital. Since I had to work during the day, my visits with dad were confined to evening hours. Regularly my golden retriever and I would drive to the nursing home to visit for a while and then return home, where I was continuing to work on my master's degree. With Bea's surgery I found myself torn between being with her and looking after my dad.

Bea's earth angels were many, and they helped alleviate my guilt at not visiting as often as I would have liked after her surgery. While Bea continued to recover and improve after her surgery, though, my dad did not. His trips to the hospital increased until he was being admitted almost every other week. I knew time was getting short and tried to spend as much time as I could with him. Hospice was called, and those folks were my earth angels. There is no more wonderful organization than hospice. The care the hospice workers provided to dad and our family was priceless.

During one hospital stay near the end of March, Dad decided it would be his last. He was tired of being stuck with needles and poked and prodded, knowing full well he was not going to get better. He had already signed a DNR for himself, and he told me he didn't want to fight his disease anymore. It was a hard conversation to have, but he spared me the burden of making that final decision in the days ahead. Dad passed away peacefully on April 8, 2009. Bea was one month into her chemo treatments at that time.

I don't have much recollection of April 2009. The death of a parent, even when it's expected, shocks the system. You function externally, but internally you live in a haze. The assault of so many emotions is exhausting. The realization that you have lost your last parent leaves you feeling very vulnerable in a way that you have never in your life felt before. Your protectors and nurturers are gone. You've lost your biggest cheerleaders in life. It forces you to live in a whole new way, and it's not an easy role to step into.

Interestingly enough, even though she was dealing with her own life-threatening disease, Bea added a nurturing role to our friendship. She understood parental loss and offered both support and comfort. In one of our e-mail correspondences, she wrote the following:

I have read your letter, and my motherly instinct just wants to hug you and say everything will be all right. Bottom line, you as well as I have the need to belong, be loved, and be cherished. Lack of worthiness, hating to let go, and finding comfort, security, and safety in the old—that's the pain I hear in your letter. I can relate to that, as it is something I have let myself face. I miss the old way of family I had thirty years ago.

This is that earthquake that shakes and breaks up the path we walk, pounded down so hard we lose sight of where we are going. Being shaken up, we are forced to really listen to the word of God. Where will I go? The upsetting of our old ways of living, thinking, being, and acting; all these trials and pains are not disasters but necessary, for us to hear the word of God, always becoming; old, but ever-new words.

How much do we want to let go is the question. The Divine Therapist allows bringing up the same thoughts and issues and the problem is the refusal to let go. It's hard to let go of something that is loved and comforting. He keeps bringing us back to the same problems until we finally let go, and then we ask, "Where are you?" and learn to listen.

You are going to be all right. I hope this makes sense, as this is something I have been pondering a lot lately. Peace, my friend.

I was out playing cards for $$$ in a game called Eighty-five and I lost my shirt. 2X, Moi.

That was Bea in a nutshell, always there with words to support and encourage, and then one last line to leave me smiling and laughing.

By early summer, things were beginning to stabilize a bit. I was adjusting to life without nursing homes and hospitals and Dad; Bea was doing well with her treatments. She was eating okay again, and we resumed our get-togethers at area restaurants, where we pondered this new path we were on. It was almost easy to slip into denial of the terminal road we were traveling.

In August I had another scare in my personal life. My beloved golden retriever, Hannah, developed a huge tumor on a middle toe of her left rear foot. She was nine years old. The vet felt sure it was cancerous and recommended amputating the toe it was growing on. The surgery was scheduled for early

September. The thought of possibly losing her and my dad in the same year, just months apart, was unbearable. If you've ever loved a dog, then you understand what I'm saying.

The surgery was successful, praise God, and Hannah made a full recovery. Within a month she was back to chasing squirrels and rabbits in the back yard. Finally, a victory over that murderous disease had been accomplished.

By mid-October, life was looking optimistic again. Hannah had recovered, Bea was finishing her treatments, and things looked stable. Bea's birthday was approaching on November 2, and we had plans to celebrate with friends. It was good to have some sense of normalcy in life again. Of course this was a new normal, one that still carried the tension of living from scan to scan, praying for a clean slate.

The holidays came and went with Bea's health still intact. Her energy ebbed and flowed, but mostly she was back to her old self. A minor car accident at Christmas was the only blip on the radar for her. We both knew the cancer was inoperable and therefore still there, but for the moment it was seemingly in remission. So, for the moment, we tentatively resumed our discussion of traveling to Bora Bora. We made no concrete plans, but it felt good just to talk about it. And it made the long, dark January nights of 2010 pass quickly as we explored the Internet sites, learning more about this island and how to get there.

Bea had a routine scope scheduled for the latter part of January 2010. It was not a pleasant thing to go through, but because she was doing so well, no one was too worried about the outcome; cautiously optimistic, but not overly worried. We were wrong.

Whether the scope stirred something up internally or the cancer had silently been marching into other organs is conjecture, but Bea began a slow downward spiral. Her eating problems returned, and by early February, she became septic and returned to the hospital. She developed problems in her kidneys and liver, which then led to having a stent inserted into her liver to drain the bile. Without the proper enzymes to digest food, her weight began to drop radically. All during February and March, she struggled, was in and out of the hospital, and had one short stay in a nursing home. During the times she was at home, she was weak, and I could visibly see the life slowly oozing out of her.

It was during one of these times at home that Bea asked me to prepare her funeral liturgy. She wanted certain readings and certain people to read; she wanted hymns that were meaningful to her to be sung. She asked me to create a memory page of her life to be printed on the back of the Mass bulletin. We spent an evening or two together with her reminiscing about her life and me taking notes. We looked through pictures, and she told me stories. Spending that time together, knowing full well the implications, was a gift, not one that I recognized at the time, but one that now helps heal my heart. It was a bittersweet moment mixed with both laughter and sorrow. Gifts sometimes come in unexpected wrappings.

I had created a few different covers for the funeral bulletin for Bea to choose from, and she ultimately chose one with a butterfly and the following words:

When we have done all the work we were sent to do on earth, we are allowed to shed our body, which imprisons our soul like a cocoon encloses a butterfly.
And when the time is right, we can let go of it and we will be free of pain, free of fears and worries, and free as a butterfly returning home to God.

The back of the funeral bulletin contained a biography of her most favorite life events, concluding with a joke about why she chose female pallbearers: the men wouldn't take her out when she was alive, so they weren't going to take her out when she was dead! Always leave them if not laughing, then at least smiling through their tears. That was Bea's motto in life and in death.

I don't think I truly appreciated Bea's inner strength during this time period. I was so overwhelmed with my own emotions during the creation of her funeral bulletin that I scarcely had room to contemplate how hard it must have been for her. It was, after all, *her* funeral bulletin. We didn't talk about it, and we both maintained a rather clinical attitude during the process. It was something that had to be done, period, and so it was. Bea gave her approval of the finished copy, and we never discussed it again.

During this same time period, Bea gave away some of her things. There were items she had that had belonged to her friend Jo, and she thought those things should go to Jo's family members, so she packed them all up and delivered them herself. She had clothes she thought were too good to be put in rummage after her death, and she personally gave them away too. She did most of this sorting and delivering during the day, while I was at work. In the evening I would get e-mails from her detailing each day's organizational divestment.

I really hated March 2010. Preparing funeral bulletins, watching Bea give away possessions, and seeing my friend's health and vitality fade renewed my anger. I didn't know where to go with it, either. Who do you get angry at? God? Cancer? Bea, for whatever irrational reason? I knew from past experience this anger was really all about me, anyway. It was my utter helplessness to stop the inevitable slide into eternity my friend was on that manifested itself in anger. It was a raw, irrational, anger so heavy with grief I could hardly breathe at times, and it was never, ever exhibited in front of Bea. We shared tears, but neither of us shared our anger. In the end, Bea claimed she had no emotions left. She was entirely spent. It was that statement from her that dissipated my anger, replacing it instead with dread and fear. It was in that moment that I knew the end was near.

The Last Days

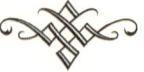

The tears fall, they're so easy to wipe off onto my sleeve,
but how do I erase the stain from my heart?
—*Unknown*

Easter weekend arrived in early April, and I had stopped by Bea's earlier in the week to bring Bea an Easter lily. Some of the flowers had not yet opened up, and she sent me e-mails each day, describing how she had literally sat and watched each one open. She was sitting a lot these days. The vomiting and dehydration were taking its toll. Her weight loss was upward of fifty pounds, and she made frequent visits to the ER for IV fluids. She so wanted to go to Easter Mass, but ended up again in the ER late Saturday night.

She came home after receiving more IV fluids, but her next week was a rough one, and she was back in the hospital again by early Saturday morning. It was April 10, and Bea was losing ground. I stopped in to visit late Saturday afternoon, and later sent this e-mail to some close friends.

Hi there,

I did go and see Bea this afternoon. She's not in very good shape. She was so very tired, and talking was such an effort. I guess Bea told her cancer doctor she didn't want to do this anymore, but he wants her to try a new type of chemo. I just didn't have the heart to push it. I told her she had to be the one to decide if she's had enough, not the doctor or any of us. I did encourage her to allow the feeding tube to be put in, though. She just can't keep throwing up like this. She has no strength left, and she needs nourishment.

I was rather shocked when she said her CA numbers were well over 2,000. Those are the cancer numbers she tells me. They were at 1,000 on Monday, and more than doubled in just a few days. That's higher than they've ever been before, much, much higher than when the cancer was discovered a year ago. That tells me the cancer is ravaging her.

I'm going to the hospital again tomorrow afternoon. I keep praying for a miracle, hoping the next time I see her, she will be better or a remission will occur. Maybe the feeding tube will renew her strength. But deep down I know there isn't much time left.

Just wanted to give you an update. Take care.

Taken from my Journal

Sunday, April 11, 2010

I went to visit Bea early this afternoon. It was a bright sunny day, and her hospital room was filled with the afternoon sun. Today we talked about her journal. She said she knew she wasn't going to be going home again, and therefore wasn't going to be writing in it anymore. It was finished. What she had written was printed out and in a folder on top of her computer desk in her bedroom. She had written her permission for me to use it on the folder cover. I was instructed to go to her home and get the folder before it got lost in the shuffle after her death. It was her final gift to me.

We talked about a lot of things today—family, friends, life, and death—all those things that make up human life. Bea seemed so peaceful today, and with the sun warming the room, it was like a moment out of time. It hardly seems possible today that she is nearing the end, but as our visit came to a close, she asked me to make the call for her to receive the Last Rites of the Church.

Monday, April 12, 2010

This has been a roller coaster day emotionally. My youngest granddaughter, Sophia Grace, was born today at 5:45 p.m. She weighed in at seven pounds, three ounces, and is 18.5 inches long. She is an absolutely beautiful baby, if I do say so myself. Courtney went into the hospital at 5:30 in the morning, already in the early stages of labor. All went well, but with little progress until around 1:00 p.m. By 5:15, Courtney was at six centimeters dilated, and from there she went very quickly to delivery at 5:45. I was able to go and see our new little family member when she was less than one hour old. What a blessing that was!

On the other hand, Bea has been in the hospital since Saturday morning with nonstop vomiting and no bowel movements for days on end. She just got two pints of blood on Friday and more fluids, but she continues to go downhill. Today they put in her feeding tube and continued to give her magnesium and potassium, in an attempt to balance her electrolytes. Her elimination is a great concern right now, and they are giving her meds in her IV to stimulate a bowel movement.

Tuesday, April 13, 2010

I went to visit Bea on my lunch hour today, and she is pretty wrung out physically and emotionally, talking about giving it all up. She is very weak, and they still haven't fed her, because they have to make sure the tube is healed enough, and right now they are still draining bile from her. I did show her pictures of my new granddaughter, which seemed to bring a little sparkle back into her eyes. The irony of new life versus fading life did not escape either of us.

After work I went to visit Courtney and Sophia and stayed until about 5:30 p.m. She was all dressed in her little pink outfit, and Courtney was dressed in her clothes too. They didn't do that back in my day until it was time to go home. We took more pictures, of course. I then went home and walked poor Hannah, who was neglected yesterday. I have to fit in schoolwork, etc., in between work and multiple hospital visits these days.

Wednesday, April 14, 2010

I visited Bea on my lunch again. Not much change, except she is still not having any bowel movements. They've tried enemas and meds in the IV, and so far no results. They had her feeding bag on but had to stop it, because she was bloating and was in great pain, because it wasn't going through. I'm not sure what they will be doing next, but she has got to have some nourishment soon, as she is literally starving to death.

I had to pick up my granddaughter, Maria, from her swimming lesson tonight so I raced home from work, walked the dog, mowed the lawn, took a shower, and grabbed something to munch on in the car. One of Bea's relatives is flying in tomorrow, and I hope that is a good thing for Bea.

Thursday, April 15, 2010

My granddaughter, Aubrey, is three years old today. She got my Little Mermaid musical card in the mail and loved it. We will celebrate her birthday on April 25, since her little sister was just born three days ago. Sophia is doing great, but Courtney is, of course, very tired.

I went to see Bea on my lunch hour again, and she was in bad shape. They had inserted a tube through her rectum and up into her intestines and gave her an enema that way today, and she was in great pain with lots of gas and cramping, but she did have elimination, finally. She has a gastrointestinal team working on her case now, so we'll see what they come up with for this problem. I'm almost afraid she will be getting a colostomy bag, but we'll see.

I'm free tonight, and the temperature is in the eighties. I put Hannah's pool out for her and did some planting and weeding. I needed a night free from running around, plus I have homework to finish.

Friday, April 16, 2010

I went to see Bea at lunchtime again today, and she is really in bad shape. They did a colonoscopy on her today and did a lot of probing around. They did find a blockage, though. Unfortunately, they didn't do anything about it and instead have her scheduled to put a stent in tomorrow. She is in such pain and moaning and saying she wants to die. She's been on morphine since last night, and why they keep putting her through this torture is making me crazy. I know it is their job to do all they can to sustain her life unless she tells them otherwise, but I can hardly stand to watch her suffer like this anymore. Part of me wishes she would die and be out of this misery. I reached this same point near the end with my mother too. The suffering is hard to bear and hard to watch. I pray God calls her home very, very soon.

Friday Evening, April 16, 2010

I went out for dinner with a friend tonight. It felt good to relax and laugh a little and talk about just ordinary life things. By evening's end, I was feeling pretty happy. That ended abruptly as soon as I answered my cell phone before I ever made it home. It was the hospital. Those people who were on the call list for Bea were asked to come to the hospital right away. Bea was dying.

Why is it that no matter how much you know the end is coming, the reality of it just slams you? I raced back to the hospital and arrived with several other friends and family members. Bea was cognizant but so weak she could only whisper. We each took our turn saying goodbye, another blessing given to us. As her breathing slowed, we gathered around her bed, laid hands on her, and sang "Peace is Flowing like a River." As we sang the final verse of Alleluias, Bea breathed her last.

Life Goes On

"I always knew looking back on my tears would bring me laughter, but I never knew looking back on my laughter would make me cry."

—*Cat Stevens*

Learning to live without someone dear to you is hard stuff. The world will give you a short amount of time to grieve, and then it expects you to get on with life. To a certain degree, it is good to keep busy as a coping mechanism, but there is no set time for grief, and everyone is different in how they deal with it. Personally, I've learned that it takes me roughly a year to fully embrace life without someone I've cared about. After my mom died, I didn't think I'd ever recover or feel happy again. Life was scary without being able to turn to her for advice and support, but then, one spring morning as I was walking the dog, I realized I was singing. I knew then that my soul had recovered, and it was going to be okay.

When my dad died, he had already been living in the nursing home for almost a year, and that grief got rolled into the grief I was carrying with me regarding Bea's cancer. There simply was no time to feel the hole that his departure left. In fact, it wasn't until Bea passed that the grief I had buried from losing my dad meshed with the grief of losing Bea. Life went on, but the emptiness their passing left me with became glaring. I spent lots of evenings in tears over the loss of so many people in my life.

It was cathartic to cry. It was also cathartic to go for long walks with my golden retriever, Hannah. Without my dad and Bea, I began to spend more time at home. Hannah and I were a team then. She missed my dad too and would sit in the doorway of his bedroom and look at me with eyes that said, "Where is he?" Hannah and I grieved together throughout that summer and into fall.

Shortly after Christmas of 2010, I learned my position at work was being eliminated. After sixteen years in this position, it was an unexpected and shocking loss. The position ended in April 2011, almost exactly one year after Bea's death in April 2010 and two years after my dad's death in April 2009. I read somewhere that the death of a loved one and the loss of a job ranked as two of the highest stressors in a person's life. In reality, it felt more like waterboarding to me, and it wasn't over yet.

The Friday before Thanksgiving 2011, Hannah and I went for our usual daily walk. We came home, had supper, and then relaxed in front of the television. We wrestled a little and played tug of war with her toy and then retired for the evening. When I awoke Saturday morning, Hannah was not on her bed in my room. I got up and found her in the hallway. Unusual, but I thought maybe she was waiting to go outside. She didn't follow me to the door. When she didn't come when I called her, I went back to see why. She hadn't moved from the hallway. I called her again, and she slowly got up, made it to the kitchen, and sank to the floor.

I knew she was in serious trouble and needed to get to a vet quickly. After lying with her on the floor for a while, I got dressed and managed to get her into the car. By the time we arrived at the vet, she could no longer walk, and they carried her in. An ultrasound showed a large splenic tumor that had ruptured. Ninety percent of splenic tumors in dogs are cancerous, and since Hannah had already had cancer once, it was more than probable that the ruptured tumor was also cancerous. Since it had ruptured already, the cancer was spilling into her abdomen. The kindest thing to do would be to put her down.

No, not my dog too! When does it end? First, my dad, then Bea, then my job, and now I was losing my beloved canine companion of eleven and a half years, Hannah. I held her in my arms and talked to her softly as the vet gave her the injection; first, the sedative to put her to sleep, and then the chemical to end her life. I stayed with her for a long time after she was gone, and they were kind enough allow me that time. I never thought I would be going home without her.

All the losses finally took their toll, and I cried for months and months. Sometimes I still cry, although time does heal all wounds. The scars remain, though, and certain things trigger memories that cause the tears to flow again.

My faith took a direct hit after Hannah died. I was finished with God. Too many losses in too short of a time span made me angry all over again at Him. I hated cancer, and I didn't know *why* God had allowed all this to happen. All those grief-laden *why* questions tumbled out of me. It took many months before I could even pray again and many more months before I could accept that God weeps with us during these times. Life is messy, and all living things will die. The joy comes in knowing we will be reunited with our loved ones in heaven.

I didn't get through all this on my own. I sought out both spiritual advice and advice from those who were trained in grief counseling. It made all the difference. The holes left by those passed on will always be a part of who I am, but so will the memories, the shared laughter, and all those other things that make up relationships. If we live long enough, we all experience loss of some kind, and one day we will be the loss that someone else will have to learn to live with. While we are here, therefore, let's love each other as best as we can, because love is really all you take with you and all you leave behind.

The refrain to one of my favorite hymns, "We Are Called," sums it up nicely.

We are called to act with justice,
We are called to love tenderly.
We are called to serve one another
And to walk humbly with God.

Pancreatic Cancer

If there ever comes a day when we can't be together
keep me in your heart, I'll stay there forever.
—*Winnie the Pooh*

New treatments for cancer are discovered every day, yet pancreatic cancer remains deadly. One of the main reasons is that the pancreas, which is an organ that secretes enzymes that aid in digestion, is virtually hidden within the body. Its very location affects the doctors' ability to see tumors and makes diagnosis harder in the earlier stages. These tumors also tend to get into areas where they are difficult to remove, such as around blood vessels and lymph nodes.

Although percentages change, depending on the stage of cancer and the treatments being used, patients with general pancreatic cancer have a life expectancy of five to eight months. Twenty percent will live at least one year, while only five percent will survive five years. My mother was told she had eight months and went on to live for four and half years. There are also people who receive an early diagnosis, like Supreme Court

Justice Ruth Bader Ginsburg, and go on to live productive lives. Every cancer journey is unique, and the number of our days, even as we are aware of the scientific data, is best left to God.

Both my mother and Bea said after their diagnoses that they knew something was wrong long before they became sick. In hindsight, there were symptoms that they wrote off as something else—heartburn, indigestion, GERD, ulcers, and on and on. Taken individually, the symptoms could indicate just about anything, but collectively, they become significant. Forewarned is forearmed, and more than two or three of the following symptoms occurring at the same time should prompt a doctor visit:

- Sudden onset diabetes with no family history
- Yellowing of the eyes or skin
- Lack of appetite
- Changes in taste
- Abdominal pain
- An enlarged gall bladder
- Pale, floating, smelly stools
- Dark, tarry stools
- Sudden, unexplained weight loss

Document all your symptoms for the doctor so he can determine the need for further tests, such as an ultrasound, a CT scan, or an endoscopy, followed by a biopsy to search for a pancreatic tumor. There is also a blood test for a biomarker called CA-19-9 that can be used in conjunction with other tests to diagnose early pancreatic cancer.

Currently pancreatic research is one of the most under-funded forms of cancer research in the United States, in spite of the fact it is the second leading cause of death in the world. Bea allowed her story to be shared with the hope that it will shed light on this deadly disease. The more people know about the grimness of the disease, perhaps the more funding pancreatic cancer research will receive. Bea's is just one voice, but together with my mother and the many other pancreatic cancer patients and survivors, their collective voices are powerful testimonies that must be heard.

www.ingramcontent.com/pod-product-compliance
Lightning Source LLC
Chambersburg PA
CBHW020356290526
45785CB00005B/2318